VISION VITALITY

Therapeutic Approaches To Eye Health

Enhance Your Vision And Eye Health With Advanced Therapies And Lifestyle Strategies For Optimal Ocular Function

DR. BRIDGET PROMISE

CHAPTER ONE

Introduction

Eye health is an important part of general well-being since our eyesight is the main way we perceive and interact with the environment.

Understanding and maintaining eye health is critical due to the eyes' complicated structure and the complexities of vision. In this examination, we will dig into the complexities of eye health, addressing the varied nature of vision and the numerous difficulties that may develop. In addition, we'll look at therapeutic ways to maintain and improve eye health, with a focus on proactive care.

Understanding Eye Health

The human eye is a wonder of biological engineering, enabling us to see a wide range of colors, fine details, and the dynamic movement of our surroundings.

It is a sophisticated sensory organ that converts light into electrical impulses, which the brain interprets as pictures. Understanding eye health is knowing the delicate balance needed for maximum performance.

Complexity Of Vision

Vision is a complicated process in which several components of the eye act in tandem. The voyage starts with the cornea and lens, which direct light to the retina. The retina comprises photoreceptor cells (rods and cones) that turn light into electrical impulses.

These impulses proceed from the optic nerve to the brain, where they are transformed into the pictures we see.

The eyes also include capabilities for adapting to changing illumination conditions. The iris controls the size of the pupil to regulate the quantity of light that enters the eye. Furthermore, ocular muscles allow us to concentrate on items from various distances.

Maintaining optimum eyesight requires a harmonious interaction of these components. Genetics, age, and environmental factors may all affect the delicate balance, resulting in frequent eye health disorders.

Common Eye Health Issues

Several common eye health disorders may affect people at all stages of life. These difficulties emerge when the eye's shape or the aging process impairs the capacity to concentrate light on the retina.

Another common worry is age-related macular degeneration (AMD), which affects the macula, the core region of the retina. AMD may cause a loss of central vision, affecting tasks such as reading and facial recognition.

Cataracts, or clouding of the eye's natural lens, often occur with age. This syndrome might result in blurred vision and sensitivity to light. Glaucoma, characterized by increasing pressure inside the eye, may damage the optic nerve and cause vision loss if not addressed.

Dry eye syndrome is a frequent problem, particularly in the digital era, when extended screen time is commonplace. This disorder develops when the eyes do not produce enough tears or the tears evaporate too rapidly, causing irritation and visual problems.

CHAPTER TWO

Exploring Therapeutic Approaches

Preserving and enhancing eye health requires a mix of preventative and treatment strategies. Regular eye examinations are critical for early diagnosis and treatment of any problems. Comprehensive eye examinations measure not just visual acuity but also the general health of the eye.

Nutrition is an essential part of maintaining eye health. Foods high in vitamins A, C, and E, as well as minerals like zinc and omega-3 fatty acids, help to improve eye function. Leafy greens, seafood, nuts, and bright fruits are examples of nutrient-dense foods that promote eye health.

Protecting the eyes from damaging ultraviolet (UV) light is critical. Wearing sunglasses with UV protection shields the eyes from the sun's damaging rays, lowering the incidence of cataracts and other UV-related problems.

Corrective lenses or contact lenses may help people with refractive problems see clearly. Advances in technology have also resulted in surgical procedures like LASIK, which reshapes the cornea to enhance vision without the need for glasses or contacts.

Treatment options for disorders like as AMD or glaucoma may include drugs, laser treatment, or surgical procedures. Early diagnosis and early care are critical for reducing the course of these diseases and maintaining eyesight.

Dry eye syndrome may typically be treated with lifestyle changes such as taking breaks during extended screen time, utilizing artificial tears, and staying hydrated. In extreme circumstances, prescription drugs may be advised.

Understanding the complexities of eye health is critical for anyone looking to maintain and improve their eyesight. The eyes, with their sophisticated structure and interaction of components, are prone to a variety of health problems. Individuals may, however, take proactive actions to preserve good eye health by getting frequent eye examinations, focusing on diet, taking precautions, and learning about new treatment options.

Incorporating these tactics into everyday life not only tackles common eye health concerns but also improves general well-being. As we traverse the world's visually rich tapestry, addressing our eye health guarantees that we can continue to enjoy the beauty and marvels that surround us.

Our eyes, sometimes regarded as the windows to the soul, play an important part in our everyday lives, molding our vision of the world. Maintaining excellent eye health is not only necessary for clear vision, but it also benefits general well-being. In addition to regular eye exams and adequate eye care practices, adopting a holistic lifestyle may have a substantial influence on eye health. This article looks at dietary methods, exercise, the influence of sleep, mindfulness techniques, and holistic ways to relieve eye strain to maintain and improve eye health.

Nutritional Strategies For Best Eye Health

A well-balanced and nutrient-dense diet is essential for general health, including good eye health. Certain nutrients are essential for maintaining eyesight and avoiding age-related eye problems.

Antioxidants such as vitamins A, C, and E, as well as minerals like zinc and omega-3 fatty acids, help to protect the eyes from oxidative damage.

1. Vitamin A: Found in carrots, sweet potatoes, and leafy greens, vitamin A is crucial for corneal health and night blindness prevention.

2. Vitamin C: Citrus fruits, strawberries, and bell peppers are high in vitamin C, which helps to avoid cataracts and promotes general eye health.

3. Vitamin E: Nuts, seeds, and spinach contain vitamin E, which

may lower the incidence of age-related macular degeneration.

4. Zinc: This mineral, found in meat, dairy, and nuts, is essential for retinal function and may help prevent AMD.

5.Omega-3 Fatty Acids: Fish, flaxseeds, and walnuts contain omega-3 fatty acids, which promote retinal health and may help prevent dry eyes.

Incorporating a variety of these nutrient-dense foods into your diet will help you maintain good eye health.

Exercise And Eye Wellness

Regular physical exercise not only improves cardiovascular health but also promotes eye health. Exercise enhances blood circulation, which is required to transport oxygen and nutrients to the eyes. In addition, physical exercise may reduce the incidence of glaucoma and AMD.

1. Cardiovascular Exercise: Walking, running, and cycling improve blood flow to the eyes, which benefits general eye health.

2. Simple eye exercises may help relieve eye strain and increase attention. Eye tiredness may be

reduced by following the 20-20-20 rule, which involves taking a 20-second break every 20 minutes to stare at anything 20 feet away.

3. Yoga for the Eyes: Certain yoga postures and eye exercises may help increase flexibility and strength in the eye muscles.

Individuals may improve their cardiovascular and ocular health by adding regular physical exercise to their daily routines.

CHAPTER THREE

The Effects Of Sleep On Vision

Quality sleep is essential for general health, and its effects extend to eye health. Inadequate or poor-quality sleep may cause eye strain, and dry eyes, and contribute to the development of diseases such as glaucoma.

1. Sleep Duration: Aim for 7-9 hours of excellent sleep each night to help your eyes to relax and regenerate.

2. Sleep Position: Sleeping on your back is often advised to lower the

risk of acquiring sleep-related eye disorders.

3. Reducing Screen Time Before Bed: Screens produce blue light, which may disturb sleep rhythms. Limit screen use at least an hour before bedtime to improve sleep quality.

Prioritizing excellent sleep hygiene improves not only general health but also the vitality of the eyes.

Mindfulness Practices For Eyecare

Mindfulness, the discipline of being present and completely involved in the present moment, may help with eye care by lowering stress and boosting relaxation.

1. Eye Relaxation Techniques: To relieve eye strain, practice palming, which involves covering your eyes with your hands, and deep breathing.

2. Mindful Breathing: Practice mindful breathing techniques to decrease general stress and improve eye health.

3. Digital detox: Take breaks from your digital gadgets and participate in mindfulness exercises like meditation to enhance relaxation and minimize eye strain.

Mindfulness activities improve not just the eyes, but also the whole well-being, improving both physical and mental health.

Holistic Approaches To Relieving Eye Strain

In today's digital era, extended screen time has become unavoidable, leading to a rise in cases of eye strain. Adopting holistic ways may assist in easing pain and preserving eye health.

1. Blinking Exercises: Consciously blink to wet the eyes and relieve dryness caused by extended screen exposure.

2. Eye Massage: Gently massaging the temples and the region surrounding the eyes helps reduce stress and enhance blood circulation.

3. Warm compresses may help relieve eye strain and relax the eye muscles.

4. Hydration: Staying hydrated promotes tear production and prevents dry eyes.

5. Adjusting Screen Settings: To decrease eye strain, put displays at eye level and adjust brightness and contrast.

These holistic techniques are simple to incorporate into everyday activities, reducing eye strain and promoting long-term eye health.

Finally, maintaining good eye health requires a holistic strategy that goes beyond typical eye care techniques. Incorporating dietary methods, regular exercise, prioritizing excellent sleep, participating in mindfulness practices, and using holistic techniques to ease eye strain all help to maintain and improve eye health. Individuals who make conscientious lifestyle choices may protect their eyes and improve long-term visual health.

Technology And Ocular Health

In today's fast-paced digital age, technology is a vital part of our everyday lives, transforming how we work, communicate, and enjoy ourselves. However, the growing dependence on digital gadgets has sparked worries about their possible influence on vision health.

From extended screen time to exposure to blue light generated by displays, our eyes confront new problems in the digital age. This article delves into several elements of technology and eye health, including designing eye-friendly workplaces, establishing critical eye care routines, researching herbal treatments for vision support, and understanding the significance of eye supplements.

CHAPTER FOUR

Eye-Friendly Workspaces

Creating an eye-friendly workstation is critical for keeping good eye health, particularly for individuals who work long hours in front of digital displays. Consider the following suggestions when designing a workstation that emphasizes your visual well-being:

1. Proper Screen Placement: To avoid neck and eye strain, position your computer screen at eye level. This guarantees that you are gazing slightly lower at the screen, which reduces discomfort.

2. Adjust Lighting: Avoid using intense overhead lighting, which might generate glare on your screen. Choose ambient lighting that evenly lights your workstation. Position your screen to reduce reflections and glare from windows or artificial light.

3. Follow the 20-20-20 Rule: To reduce eye strain, use the 20-20-20 rule. Every 20 minutes, take a 20-second break and stare 20 feet away. This simple activity helps to alleviate eye strain induced by extended screen use.

4. Use Blue Light Filters: Digital displays generate blue light, which

may disturb sleep patterns and cause eye strain. Consider using blue light filters or glasses intended to lessen the effects of blue light on your eyes, particularly in the evening.

5. Blink often: Staring at screens often leads to less blinking, resulting in dry eyes. Make a deliberate effort to blink often to keep your eyes moist and limit the possibility of pain.

Essential Eye Care Habits

In addition to improving your workstation, practicing good eye care routines will help you maintain your vision in the long run. Include the following routines in your routine to help your eyes:

1. Stay Hydrated: Adequate hydration is critical for general health, including eye health. Drink plenty of water to keep your eyes moist and lubricated.

2. Maintain a Balanced Diet: Nutrient-dense meals improve eye health. Consume meals rich in vitamins A, C, and E, as well as zinc and omega-3 fatty acids. Leafy greens, seafood, nuts, and bright fruits are all great options for boosting your eyesight.

3. Regular eye exams are essential for spotting any problems early

on. Even if you don't have visual difficulties, frequent check-ups may help you maintain your eye health and catch problems before they become severe.

4. Protect Your Eyes from UV radiation: Prolonged exposure to the sun's ultraviolet (UV) radiation may cause cataracts and other eye problems. To protect your eyes from dangerous rays, use UV-protective sunglasses while you are outside.

5. Practice the 20-20-20 guideline Outside of Work: Apply the 20-20-20 guideline to various areas of your life. Take pauses when

reading a book, doing housework, or indulging in hobbies to rest your eyes and lessen strain.

Herbal Solutions For Vision Support

For millennia, numerous civilizations have used herbal medicines to promote eye health. While these cures are not a replacement for expert medical advice, certain plants are thought to improve eyesight. Before adopting the following herbal choices into your regimen, use caution and check with a healthcare practitioner.

1.   Bilberry: Known   for   its antioxidant   characteristics, bilberry is said to improve night vision and general eye health. It is available as a supplement, but the dose should be reviewed with a healthcare professional.

2. Ginkgo biloba is well known for its possible cognitive advantages, but it may also have a good impact on eye health. It is claimed to enhance blood flow to the eyes and prevent   age-related   macular degeneration.

3. Eyebright has traditionally been used in herbal therapy to relieve eye irritation and inflammation. It

is available in a variety of formats, including teas and supplements.

4. Turmeric: With its anti-inflammatory characteristics, turmeric is gaining popularity for its potential benefits to eye health. Curcumin, turmeric's main ingredient, is being investigated for its potential involvement in the prevention and treatment of eye problems.

Understanding Eye Supplements

Many people use eye supplements to maintain good eye health. These supplements often include a mix of vitamins, minerals, and antioxidants designed particularly to improve eyesight. However, you must approach eye supplements with an awareness of their intended purpose and possible advantages.

1. Vitamin A is essential for sustaining healthy eyesight and plays an important role in retinal function. While vitamin A deficiency may cause visual difficulties, excessive consumption should be avoided since it might have negative consequences.

2. Vitamin C and E: These antioxidants protect the eyes from oxidative damage. Vitamin C

strengthens blood vessels in the eyes, but vitamin E may lower the risk of age-related macular degeneration.

3. Lutein and zeaxanthin: High concentrations of these carotenoids in the retina have been linked to a decreased incidence of age-related macular degeneration and cataracts. They are typically found in eye supplements.

4.Omega-3 Fatty Acids: Found in fish oil supplements, omega-3 fatty acids improve general eye health and may lower the risk of dry eyes and macular degeneration.

While eye supplements might be useful, it is important to contact a healthcare expert before incorporating them into your regimen. Nutrient requirements differ from person to person, and taking too much of some vitamins and minerals may be harmful. Furthermore, optimal eye health is built on a well-balanced diet rich in critical nutrients.

Finally, as technology advances, it becomes more important to address eye health in our everyday lives. Individuals may take proactive actions to protect their eyesight in the digital era by building eye-friendly workplaces, adopting fundamental eye care practices, exercising caution while investigating herbal cures, and understanding the function of eye supplements.

Regular eye exams, a balanced lifestyle, and a conscious attitude to technology usage all help to keep eyes healthy for years to come.

CHAPTER FIVE

Vision Therapy Techniques: Enhancing Eye Health Naturally

In a society dominated by screens and continual visual stimulation, the health of our eyes is sometimes overlooked. Vision therapy approaches provide a comprehensive approach to organically treating eye disorders, emphasizing the complex relationship between our visual well-being and general health. As we study vision therapy, we will look at the many approaches available, the influence of stress on vision disorders, and preventative strategies for long-term eye health.

Vision therapy is a specialist kind of rehabilitation that focuses on improving and managing visual function. Unlike traditional therapies that depend mainly on corrective lenses or surgery, vision therapy takes a more holistic approach, treating the root causes of visual problems.

This treatment technique consists of a series of exercises and activities aimed at improving visual skills such as eye movement, coordination, and concentration ability.

Various vision therapy procedures are used to address a broad variety of visual difficulties. One popular approach is eye-tracking exercises. These workouts include following a moving object with your eyes, which improves coordination and tracking ability. Individuals who suffer from conditions such as lazy eyes or difficulty reading may find these exercises very effective in retraining their eyes to operate together flawlessly.

Convergence exercises are also an important part of vision rehabilitation. Convergence is the capacity of the eyes to move together when focusing on a close object. When this capacity is weakened, it may cause eye strain, double vision, and difficulty maintaining concentration. Convergence exercises attempt to strengthen the eye muscles that bring the eyes together, resulting in greater coordination.

Accommodation exercises are also very important in vision treatment. Accommodation refers to the eyes' capacity to shift focus from close to great distances. Prolonged screen time and close-up work may often cause a loss in this skill. Individuals who do accommodation exercises may improve their eye flexibility and lessen the chance of pain associated with extended close employment.

Stress And Vision Problems

Stress, an unavoidable component of contemporary life, may have a substantial influence on our general health, including our eyesight. The relationship between stress and vision difficulties is complex, with stress appearing both directly and indirectly in a variety of ocular diseases. Understanding this link is critical for taking a comprehensive approach to eye care.

Visual stress is a direct consequence of stress on vision. This illness may cause symptoms including impaired vision, light sensitivity, and headaches. Visual stress is especially frequent among those who spend a lot of time in front of screens, which leads to a condition known as computer vision syndrome (CVS). Prolonged screen exposure stresses the eyes, causing pain and visual problems.

Stress may indirectly increase pre-existing problems like dry eye syndrome. Stress causes physiological reactions in the body, including reduced tear production. This decrease might result in dry, inflamed eyes, which reduces visual comfort. Furthermore, persistent stress may lead to disorders such as glaucoma and macular degeneration, highlighting the need for stress management in long-term eye health.

Preventive Strategies For Long-Term Eye Health

While vision therapy approaches may help with current visual problems, preventative steps are also important for sustaining long-term eye health. Incorporating these strategies throughout everyday life may improve general health and lessen the likelihood of acquiring visual difficulties.

1. Follow the 20-20-20 rule to reduce the negative impacts of excessive screen usage. Every 20 minutes, take a 20-second break and stare 20 feet away. This technique reduces eye strain and encourages better visual habits.

2. Maintain a balanced diet: Proper nutrition is essential for eye health. Incorporate foods high in vitamins and minerals, especially those that are good for your eyes, such as vitamins A, C, and E, as well as lutein and

zeaxanthin. Leafy vegetables, carrots, and seafood are all great alternatives.

3. Stay hydrated: Proper hydration promotes general health, including eye health. Dehydration may add to dry eye problems, so drink plenty of water throughout the day.

4. Protect your eyes from UV rays, since prolonged exposure may lead to cataracts and other eye disorders. Wear sunglasses that filter both UVA and UVB radiation while going outside, especially on overcast days.

5. Practice proper lighting habits: When doing close-up work, be sure to use suitable lighting. Avoid glare from overhead lights or windows, and adjust your computer screen to reduce reflections. A well-lit office alleviates eye strain.

6. Get frequent eye exams: Routine eye exams are critical for early diagnosis of any problems. Regular check-ups provide proactive management and intervention, therefore avoiding the advancement of some eye problems.

Conclusion

In the field of vision therapy, a more holistic approach to eye health is emerging, going beyond the conventional dependence on corrective lenses and surgical procedures. Vision therapy procedures allow people to actively engage in enhancing their visual abilities and treating underlying difficulties. Furthermore, acknowledging the role of stress in vision disorders highlights the need for stress management in maintaining good eye health.

By incorporating preventative measures into our everyday lives, we empower ourselves to protect our eyesight in the long run. The 20-20-20 rule, a balanced diet, enough hydration, UV protection, excellent lighting practices, and frequent eye exams all contribute to a comprehensive approach to eye care.

In a world where our eyes are continuously inundated with stimuli, taking proactive actions to protect our eyesight is critical. Vision therapy approaches, together with stress management and preventative measures, pave the way for a future in which excellent eye health is not only a goal but a long-term reality.

THYROID THERAPY GUIDE

Treatment For Balancing Hormones And Energy Levels

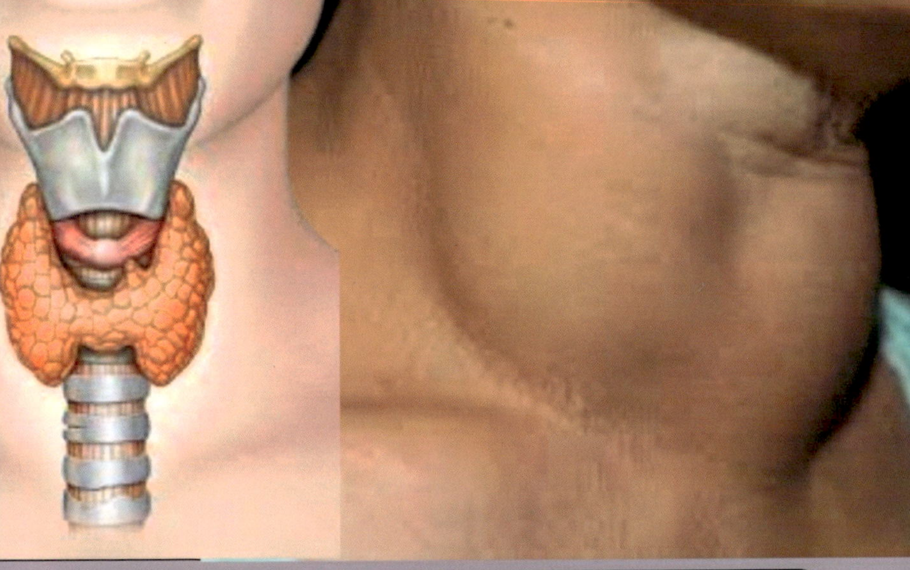

Fine-Tune Your Thyroid Function With Therapies That Balance Hormones And Boost Overall Energy Levels

DR. BRIDGET PROMISE